TOOTH DECAY

Symptoms, Causes, Treatment, and Prevention

Patrick Odega

Dedication

To my beloved Mother,

Thank you for being my guiding light and unwavering support throughout my life. Your selflessness, kindness, and unconditional love have been the foundation of my being.

I dedicate my accomplishments and successes to you, knowing that they would not have been possible without your guidance and encouragement. Your unwavering faith in me has been a constant source of motivation, and I am grateful for your sacrifices and endless efforts to make me the person I am today.

You have always been there for me, through the good times and the bad. Your strength, resilience, and wisdom have been my inspiration, and I am honored to have you as my mother.

I dedicate this to you as a small token of my appreciation, with the hope that it will bring a smile to your face and warmth to your heart. Thank you for everything, Mom. I love you more than words can express.

With Love,

Patrick

Table Of Contents

6.2 Final Thoughts

Chapter1:

Introduction

Tooth decay, also known as dental caries or cavities, is a common dental problem that occurs when bacteria in the mouth produce acids that attack the tooth enamel. This acid can gradually dissolve the enamel, causing small holes or cavities to form in the teeth. If left untreated, tooth decay can progress and affect the deeper layers of the tooth, leading to tooth sensitivity, pain, and even tooth loss. Tooth decay is a preventable condition, and maintaining good oral hygiene practices, a healthy diet, and regular dental check-ups can help prevent it.

The bacteria that cause tooth decay thrives on sugars and carbohydrates found in foods and drinks, which they convert into acid. If the acid is allowed to remain on the tooth surface, it can lead to demineralization of the enamel, making it weaker and more susceptible to decay.

Tooth decay can occur in anyone, regardless of age, but it is most common in children and teenagers. Other risk factors include poor oral hygiene, dry mouth, certain medical conditions, and genetic factors.

The symptoms of tooth decay may vary depending on the severity and location of the decay. In the early stages, there may be no symptoms at all, but as the decay progresses, common symptoms include tooth sensitivity, pain when eating or drinking, visible holes or discoloration on teeth, and bad breath.

Treatment for tooth decay depends on the extent of the decay and can range from fillings and crowns to root canal treatment and tooth extraction. The goal of treatment is to remove the decay and restore the affected tooth's structure and function.

Prevention is key to avoiding tooth decay. This can be achieved by maintaining good oral hygiene practices, such as brushing teeth twice a day, flossing daily, and using mouthwash. Additionally, eating a balanced diet that limits sugary and acidic foods and beverages and regularly visiting the dentist for check-ups and cleanings can help prevent tooth decay.

Tooth decay is a common dental problem that can lead to significant pain and discomfort if left untreated. Fortunately, it is a preventable condition, and simple lifestyle changes and regular dental check-ups can help prevent and treat it.

Understanding tooth decay is crucial for maintaining good oral health and preventing dental problems. Tooth decay is a common dental problem that affects people of all ages, and it can lead to significant pain, discomfort, and even tooth loss if left untreated.

By understanding the causes and risk factors of tooth decay, individuals can take steps to prevent it. Maintaining good oral hygiene practices, such as brushing teeth twice a day, flossing daily, and using mouthwash, can help remove plaque and bacteria from the mouth, preventing the buildup of acids that can lead to tooth decay.

A healthy diet that is low in sugary and acidic foods and beverages can also help prevent tooth decay. Regular dental check-ups and cleanings are also essential for identifying and treating tooth decay early, before it progresses and causes significant damage to the teeth.

Moreover, understanding tooth decay can also help individuals recognize the early symptoms of the condition, such as tooth sensitivity and pain when eating or drinking, and seek prompt treatment to prevent further damage.

In summary, understanding tooth decay is critical for maintaining good oral health and preventing dental problems. By taking simple steps to prevent tooth decay and seeking prompt treatment, individuals can maintain healthy teeth and gums and avoid significant pain, discomfort, and tooth loss.

Chapter2:

Symptoms of Tooth Decay

Tooth sensitivity- Is a common dental problem that affects many people. It is characterized by a sudden, sharp pain or discomfort in one or more teeth when exposed to certain stimuli, such as hot or cold foods and drinks, sweet or sour foods, and cold air.

Tooth sensitivity occurs when the protective layer of enamel that covers the teeth becomes worn down or eroded, exposing the underlying dentin layer. The dentin layer contains tiny tubules that lead to the nerve endings of the tooth, and when these tubules are exposed to external stimuli, it can cause pain or discomfort.

There are several factors that can contribute to tooth sensitivity, including:

1. **Brushing too hard:** Brushing the teeth too hard or using a hard-bristled toothbrush can wear down the enamel, exposing the dentin layer and causing sensitivity.

2. **Gum recession:** Gum recession can occur as a result of gum disease, age, or aggressive brushing, and it can expose the roots of the teeth, which are more sensitive than the enamel.

3. **Tooth decay:** Tooth decay can weaken the enamel and expose the dentin layer, leading to sensitivity.

4. **Teeth grinding:** Grinding or clenching the teeth can wear down the enamel and cause sensitivity.

5. **Acidic foods and drinks:**
   Consuming acidic foods and
   drinks, such as citrus fruits and
   soda, can erode the enamel and
   expose the dentin layer.
6. **Dental procedures:** Certain
   dental procedures, such as teeth
   whitening and dental fillings, can
   cause temporary sensitivity.

Treatment for tooth sensitivity depends
on the underlying cause. In some cases,
using a desensitizing toothpaste or
applying a fluoride gel or varnish to the
teeth can help reduce sensitivity. Other
treatments may include filling cavities or
treating gum disease to reduce gum
recession, using a mouthguard to
prevent teeth grinding, or avoiding
acidic foods and drinks.

In summary, tooth sensitivity is a
common dental problem that can cause
significant pain and discomfort.
Understanding the causes and risk

factors of tooth sensitivity can help individuals take steps to prevent it, and seeking prompt treatment can help reduce symptoms and improve oral health.

Pain when Eating or Drinking- Experiencing pain or discomfort when eating or drinking can be a sign of a dental problem, and it is important to seek prompt treatment to prevent further damage to the teeth.

There are several possible causes of pain when eating or drinking, including:

1. Tooth decay: Tooth decay can cause pain or discomfort when eating or drinking sweet or acidic foods and drinks, as the decay weakens the enamel and exposes

the sensitive dentin layer of the tooth.

2. Cracked or fractured teeth: A cracked or fractured tooth can cause pain or discomfort when eating or drinking, especially when biting down on hard foods.

3. Gum disease: Gum disease can cause pain or discomfort when eating or drinking, especially if the gums are inflamed or infected.

4. Tooth abscess: A tooth abscess is a pocket of pus that can form inside the tooth or in the gum tissue, and it can cause severe pain when eating or drinking.

5. Sensitivity: Tooth sensitivity, which is caused by the exposure of the dentin layer of the tooth, can cause pain or discomfort when eating or drinking hot or cold foods and drinks.

Treatment for pain when eating or drinking depends on the underlying cause. In some cases, using a desensitizing toothpaste or applying a fluoride gel or varnish to the teeth can help reduce sensitivity. Other treatments may include filling cavities, placing a dental crown or bridge to repair a cracked or fractured tooth, treating gum disease, or performing a root canal to treat a tooth abscess.

Prevention is key to avoiding pain when eating or drinking. Maintaining good oral hygiene practices, such as brushing teeth twice a day, flossing daily, and using mouthwash, can help prevent tooth decay and gum disease. Additionally, avoiding sugary and acidic foods and drinks, wearing a mouth guard to protect teeth from injury during sports or other activities, and visiting the dentist regularly for check-ups and cleanings can help prevent dental problems and reduce the risk of pain when eating or drinking.

In summary, experiencing pain or discomfort when eating or drinking can be a sign of a dental problem, and it is important to seek prompt treatment to prevent further damage to the teeth. Understanding the causes and risk factors of pain when eating or drinking can help individuals take steps to prevent it, and seeking prompt treatment can help reduce symptoms and improve oral health.

Visible Holes or Discoloration on Teeth- Visible holes or discoloration on teeth are signs of tooth decay or cavities. Tooth decay is a common dental problem that occurs when bacteria in the mouth produce acid that eats away at the tooth's enamel and creates a hole or cavity.

In the early stages of tooth decay, there may be no visible signs or symptoms. However, as the decay progresses, visible holes or discoloration may appear on the teeth. These may appear as dark spots or stains on the surface of the tooth, or as pits or craters that can be felt with the tongue.

Tooth decay can also cause sensitivity to hot or cold foods and drinks, and may cause pain or discomfort when biting down or chewing. If left untreated, tooth decay can lead to further complications, such as tooth infection, abscesses, and tooth loss.

Treatment for visible holes or discoloration on teeth depends on the extent of the decay. In the early stages of tooth decay, a dentist may recommend a fluoride treatment or dental filling to repair the cavity and prevent further decay. If the decay has progressed further, a root canal or tooth extraction may be necessary to remove the infected tooth.

Prevention is key to avoiding visible holes or discoloration on teeth. Maintaining good oral hygiene practices, such as brushing teeth twice a day, flossing daily, and using mouthwash, can help prevent tooth decay. Additionally, avoiding sugary and acidic foods and drinks, wearing a mouth guard to protect teeth from injury during sports or other activities, and visiting the dentist regularly for check-ups and cleanings can help prevent dental problems and reduce the risk of visible holes or discoloration on teeth.

In summary, visible holes or discoloration on teeth are signs of tooth decay or cavities, which can lead to further complications if left untreated. Understanding the causes and risk factors of tooth decay can help individuals take steps to prevent it, and seeking prompt treatment can help reduce symptoms and improve oral health.

Bad breath- Bad breath, also known as halitosis, is a common dental problem that can be embarrassing and uncomfortable. Bad breath is often caused by poor oral hygiene practices, but it can also be a sign of other underlying dental or medical conditions.

The most common cause of bad breath is poor oral hygiene practices, such as not brushing and flossing regularly, which can lead to the buildup of bacteria and food particles in the mouth. This bacteria can produce sulfur compounds that create an unpleasant odor.

Other possible causes of bad breath include gum disease, dry mouth, smoking, certain medications, and medical conditions such as sinus infections, acid reflux, and diabetes.

Treatment for bad breath depends on the underlying cause. In many cases, improving oral hygiene practices, such as brushing and flossing regularly, using mouthwash, and cleaning the tongue, can help reduce bad breath. If the bad breath is caused by gum disease or other dental issues, treatment may involve deep cleaning, antibiotics, or other dental procedures.

For individuals with chronic bad breath caused by medical conditions, such as acid reflux or diabetes, treating the underlying condition can help reduce bad breath.

Prevention is key to avoiding bad breath. Maintaining good oral hygiene practices, such as brushing teeth twice a day, flossing daily, and using mouthwash, can help prevent the buildup of bacteria and food particles in the mouth. Additionally, avoiding tobacco products, staying hydrated to prevent dry mouth, and visiting the dentist regularly for check-ups and cleanings can help prevent dental problems and reduce the risk of bad breath.

In summary, bad breath is a common dental problem that can be caused by poor oral hygiene practices, dental issues, or underlying medical conditions. Understanding the causes and risk factors of bad breath can help individuals take steps to prevent it, and seeking prompt treatment can help reduce symptoms and improve oral health.

Chapter3:

Causes of Tooth Decay

Tooth decay is caused by a combination of factors that create an environment in the mouth where bacteria can thrive and produce acid. The following are some of the most common causes of tooth decay:

Poor oral hygiene: When individuals do not brush and floss their teeth regularly, food particles and bacteria can build up on the teeth, leading to the formation of plaque. Plaque produces acid that can erode the tooth's enamel, leading to decay.

High-sugar diet: Consuming foods and drinks that are high in sugar can increase the amount of acid in the mouth and create an environment that is conducive to tooth decay.

Acidic foods and drinks: Consuming foods and drinks that are high in acid, such as citrus fruits, soda, and sports drinks, can erode the tooth's enamel and increase the risk of decay.

Dry mouth: Saliva helps to neutralize acid in the mouth and wash away food particles and bacteria. When the mouth is dry, either due to medication or a medical condition, the risk of tooth decay increases.

Genetics: Some individuals may be more prone to tooth decay due to their genetics. For example, some people may have weaker tooth enamel, making their teeth more susceptible to decay.

Age: As individuals age, their teeth may become more vulnerable to decay due to wear and tear, receding gums, and other age-related factors.

Dental problems: If an individual has a cracked or chipped tooth, or if they have a dental filling or crown that has become damaged, bacteria can enter the tooth and cause decay.

Understanding the causes of tooth decay can help individuals take steps to prevent it. Maintaining good oral hygiene practices, consuming a healthy diet, and visiting the dentist regularly for check-ups and cleanings can help prevent dental problems and reduce the risk of tooth decay.

Chapter4:

Treatment of Tooth Decay

The treatment of tooth decay depends on the severity of the decay and the extent of damage to the tooth. In its early stages, tooth decay may be treated with simple interventions such as fluoride treatments and improved oral hygiene practices. However, if left untreated, tooth decay can progress and cause more serious problems that may require more extensive treatment.

The following are some common treatments for tooth decay:

Fillings: If the decay has not reached the pulp of the tooth, a dental filling can be used to restore the tooth. The decayed area of the tooth is removed, and the cavity is filled with a material such as composite resin, amalgam, or gold.

Root canal therapy: If the decay has reached the pulp of the tooth, a root canal may be necessary. During a root canal, the dentist removes the infected pulp, cleans and disinfects the root canal, and fills the space with a material to prevent further infection.

Crowns: If the decay has caused extensive damage to the tooth, a dental crown may be needed. A crown is a cap that is placed over the damaged tooth to restore its shape and function.

Extraction: In cases where the tooth decay is so severe that it cannot be saved with other treatments, the tooth may need to be extracted.

To avoiding tooth decay and the need for extensive dental treatment. Maintaining good oral hygiene practices, such as brushing teeth twice a day, flossing daily, and using mouthwash, can help prevent the buildup of bacteria and food particles in the mouth.

Additionally, consuming a healthy diet, avoiding sugary and acidic foods and drinks, and visiting the dentist regularly for check-ups and cleanings can help prevent dental problems and reduce the risk of tooth decay.

Chapter5:

Prevention of Tooth Decay

Preventing tooth decay is important in maintaining good oral health and avoiding dental problems.

Here are some tips to help prevent tooth decay:

Practice good oral hygiene: Brushing your teeth twice a day with fluoride toothpaste and flossing daily can help remove food particles and bacteria from your mouth, reducing the risk of tooth decay.

Use fluoride products: Fluoride helps strengthen tooth enamel, making it more resistant to decay. Using fluoride toothpaste, mouthwash, and getting professional fluoride treatments from your dentist can help prevent tooth decay.

Limit sugary and acidic foods and drinks: Consuming sugary and acidic foods and drinks can increase the amount of acid in your mouth and contribute to tooth decay. Limiting these foods and drinks can help reduce your risk of developing tooth decay.

Chew sugar-free gum: Chewing sugar-free gum after meals can help stimulate saliva production, which can neutralize acid in the mouth and wash away food particles.

Drink plenty of water: Drinking water can help wash away food particles and bacteria from your mouth and keep your mouth hydrated, which can reduce your risk of tooth decay.

Visit the dentist regularly: Regular dental check-ups and cleanings can help detect early signs of tooth decay and other dental problems, and professional cleaning can remove plaque and tartar buildup that cannot be removed with regular brushing and flossing.

By following these tips, you can help prevent tooth decay and maintain good oral health.

Chapter6:

Conclusion

Tooth decay is a common dental problem that can lead to pain, sensitivity, and other dental complications if left untreated. Understanding the symptoms, causes, treatment, and prevention of tooth decay is crucial in maintaining good oral health.

Early detection and treatment of tooth decay can prevent the need for more extensive dental procedures, such as root canals or extractions.

Good oral hygiene practices, such as brushing, flossing, and using fluoride products, along with a healthy diet and regular dental check-ups, can help prevent tooth decay.

In conclusion, by taking care of your teeth and practicing good oral hygiene habits, you can prevent tooth decay and maintain a healthy smile for years to come.

Regular visits to the dentist and early detection of dental problems can help ensure that any issues are addressed promptly, helping to prevent more serious dental problems down the road.

www.ingramcontent.com/pod-product-compliance
Lightning Source LLC
Chambersburg PA
CBHW071124220526
45467CB00004B/2039